# The Story of

# *Bella*

## By Allen "Buddy" Shuh

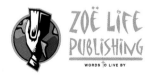

ZOË LIFE PUBLISHING

WORDS TO LIVE BY

Published by:

Zoë Life Publishing

P.O. Box 871066

Canton, MI 48187 USA

www.zoelifepub.com

All scripture quotations, unless otherwise indicated, are taken from The New King James Version (NKJV) of the Bible Copyright © 1982 by Thomas Nelson, Inc. The Bible text designated (RSV) is from the Revised Standard Version of The Bible, Copyright © 1946, 1952, 1971 by the Division of Christian Education of the National Council of the Churches of Christ in the USA. The Bible text designated (TLB) is from The Living Bible Copyright © 1971 by Tyndale House Publishers, Inc. Scripture quotations marked (NIV) are taken from the Holy Bible, New International Version ®. Copyright © 1973, 1978, 1984 by International Bible Society. Scripture quotations marked as (NLT) are taken from the New Living Translation Holy Bible. New Living Translation copyright © 1996 by Tyndale Charitable Trust. Scripture quotations marked as (NASB) are taken from the New American Standard Bible Copyright © 1960, 1962, 1963, 1968, 1971, 1972, 1973, 1975, 1977, 1995 by The Lockman Foundation. The Bible text designated (MSG) is from The Message Bible Copyright © 1993, 1994, 1995, 1996, 2000, 2001, 2002 by Eugene H. Peterson.

Take note that the name satan and associated names are not capitalized. We choose not to give him any preeminence, even to the point of violating grammatical rules.

Author:            Allen Shuh

Cover Design:      Chamira Jones

Editor:            Eastla Smith

First U.S. Edition 2006

For current information about releases by Allen Shuh or other releases from Zoë Life Publishing, visit our Web site: http://www.zoelifepub.com

Printed in the United States of America

# V2 11 28 06

# Dedication

As I sit trying to think of all the people who helped me write this book, or ran to help me in times of trouble, I find there are too many names to mention. This book is as much about those unsung heroes as it is about my experiences with my daughter. If you are one of those, and you know who you are, thank you. With that in mind, I'd like to single one person out.

I dedicate this book to my wife, Shelby Christine Shuh. Shelby, you are the most amazing person I've ever met. We went through the fire together, and you made all the difference for me. You inspired me with your love for your daughter. Whenever I think of you rocking our little girl, singing to her and praying over her, I begin to cry and wonder what I ever did to deserve such a perfect woman. Even though you were going through the worst thing imaginable, you were sensitive to me and always trying to make sure I was doing okay too. How could you be so unselfish? When I needed space, you seemed to sense it and let me go off by myself and lose myself in Sudoku puzzles so I would not have to deal with the pain. When I needed to talk, we would sit and talk and cry together. You are the best friend I've ever had and I don't know what it would have been like to go through this without you. I love you more than you know.

*-Buddy*

# The Story of

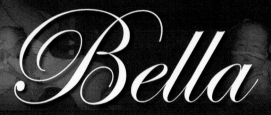

# Bella

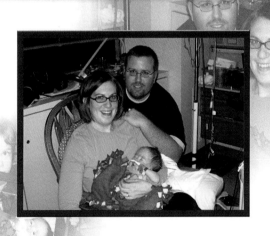

## By Allen "Buddy" Shuh

# Table of Contents

# Foreword

I have known the author, Allen "Buddy" Shuh, for most of my life. He is a mentor, a counselor, and a friend. I have always looked to him for advice and as an example. He has taught me countless lessons in the classroom, church services, and in living rooms where we have had countless conversations about life, God, and how to live like Christ. Through this story I saw him live the lessons that he had been teaching me for years. I saw his character shine through the hard situations he was facing. He was an example for anyone facing the difficulties that life sends our ways, and he would be the first to admit that it is only because his example was Christ. He was faced with death, and he looked to God for life. His story, as heartbreaking as it is, is a story of hope and faith. It is a story of how even through dark times, God's light shines through.

Throughout my life I have always been very possessive of those that I find important. I always wondered why others did not place the same value on certain people as I did. I realized that it is because people place importance on those that have impacted their lives in a great way. This being the case, Isabella Harmony Shuh is one of the most important people I have ever met. Watching her fight daily was the most inspirational thing I have ever witnessed. I asked myself many times, why do people die? It is not until I met Bella that I learned the answer to this question: it is to make life important. I have heard people say, "What a shame that she died. She did not get to live a full life." I wonder, is that true? Most people would equate a "full life" with the accumulation of things and accomplishments. It is my opinion that a full life is a life lived to impact those around us. That was Bella's life. Because of this beautiful baby girl, my life and many others will never be the same. I cannot waste the time I have been given. I must impact others with the life I have. I learned more about faith and love from her life and death, than any preacher has ever taught me. If you find yourself in the midst of a hard situation, read this book and find hope. Know that even in the face of defeat we have victory.

This story is a beautiful description of how God always has us in His arms. He is always concerned about us and loves us through everything. We can always have hope in the thought that no matter what, God loves us unconditionally. He knows our pain and He hurts with us, but He knows that death is not the end, but the beginning of a greater existence. One day I will see Bella again, and until then I have to put to use the lessons that she taught me, live life to the fullest and impact others, or else you are just a *"greedy little pig."*

*- Joel Hays*
*College student and close friend*

# Introduction:
## The Picture *"Almost"* Perfect Life

*White picket fences. 2.3 children. A nice car, a great job, the perfect home. These were some of the things you always imagined would be in your life. Me too.*

YOU WERE WELL on your way. You had many great things and it was looking like the fairy tale that you pictured. Then "it" happened.

"It" is different for different people. You might have been fired from your job. Or maybe for you, it was a divorce. You thought your husband was perfect and then he hit you. Or maybe someone you knew died unexpectedly.

Whatever "it" is, at some point you found out that not every event in life happens as you would have planned it. You have encountered tough times that you did not foresee.

What do we do when "it" happens? How do we deal with those painful times in life? I offer you my story, my pain, my life. In sharing with you, my hope is that we both will be better off because of it.

My daughter, Isabella Harmony Shuh, died on March 8th, 2006. There you have it. Yes, this is a book about hope, but I don't want to mislead you into thinking everything turns out perfect in the end. This is not a fictional movie where you know the end will be a great reversal of fortunes. This story has its ups and downs, like anyone's real life story, and has both a sad and a happy ending, depending on your outlook on life.

Throughout our ordeal, my wife and I have read many books about miracles, and they were a great encouragement to us. We did not, however, find many books written in the midst of pain and suffering that gave keen insight into how to still hope and see God when it hurts so badly. I am writing this book in the hope that it will help someone who has been wounded but wants to carry on.

*There's more to come: We continue*
*to shout our praise even when we're*
*hemmed in with troubles, because*
*we know how troubles can develop*
*passionate patience in us, and how that*
*patience in turn forges the tempered*
*steel of virtue, keeping us alert for*
*whatever God will do next. In alert*
*expectancy such as this, we're never*
*left feeling shortchanged. Quite the*
*contrary—we can't round up enough*
*containers to hold everything God*
*generously pours into our lives through*
*the Holy Spirit!*
-Romans 5:3-5 (MSG)

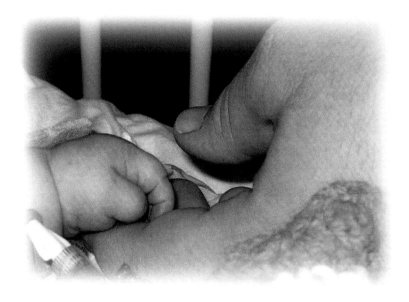

*Bella and Cousin Allen Rodriguez's fingers touch*

# 1

## First Sight
## "First Ultrasound"

*People have differing opinions on the subject of finding out a baby's gender prior to birth. Some want the surprise on the baby's birthday. Others want to prep the nursery. Me: I just want to know because I think it's cool either way.*

I WAS VERY excited to get the results of the ultrasound. My wife was almost 19 weeks pregnant. We were about to chaperone a senior class trip for the school that I work at, so we would not be in town when she hit the 20-week mark. We opted to have the ultrasound a week early rather than a week late.

I was excited because I remembered the first time I went for this ultrasound with our son, Isaac. At that time, I had stated that I didn't prefer a boy or girl, and I think I was being truthful. Yet when I found out that we were having a boy, something overwhelmed me and I started to cry.

At the time, I couldn't ascertain why I was emotional, but now I have some insights. It seems to me that discovering the gender of your child is a step in the direction of discovering the wonder that is your child. It was the same sort of thing when I saw the images of the ultrasound. I was starting to get to know my son.

So it happened again, just like the first time. I was giddy and did not really care what the gender of my child was. Part of me wanted a little boy so my son would have a male playmate, and another part of me really wanted to have a girl.

We went in and the ultrasound began. I had no clue how they could decipher what was what. To me, everything looked the same. It was all blobs of black and white. The only thing I did notice was that the procedure was taking longer than last time and the nurse seemed to be in a bad mood.

After a while, I couldn't wait anymore. I asked the nurse if she could determine our baby's gender. She told me that she thought it was a girl. Thought? I was no expert, but it seemed to me that there was a surefire way to find out. After a while longer, I asked the nurse how sure she was. She told me she was 75 percent sure. Good enough for me. It was a girl and I was thrilled!

The nurse told us that she needed us to wait in the waiting room. While waiting, I began calling our family and friends to give them the good news. I also sent two text messages to two members of our youth group. One message I sent because my wife and I are close with the youth's family, and the other I sent because I was supposed to be helping coach a softball game and was now going to be late. The significance of these two messages will become clearer in the next chapter.

As we sat in the waiting room, I noticed that my wife looked rather upset. I wondered why she wasn't happy like I was, and she told me that she didn't like that we had to wait like we were. She thought that something was up. I've come to discover that women are much more perceptive than men when it comes to certain things. I was clueless.

A short while later, the nurse came in. She told us that there was some bad news, but regulations forbade her from telling us. There was another nurse holding a phone, and she told us there was someone on the line who would tell us more.

I looked into my wife's eyes and I saw that she was about to crumble. I took the phone and talked to a doctor. What the doctor told me made me want to vomit. From that phone call and moving forward, life would never be the same for me.

*Oh yes, you shaped me first inside, then out; you formed me in my mother's womb. I thank you, High God—you're breathtaking! Body and soul, I am marvelously made! I worship in adoration—what a creation! You know me inside and out, you know every bone in my body; you know exactly how I was made, bit by bit, how I was sculpted from nothing into something. Like an open book, you watched me grow from conception to birth;   all the stages of my life were spread out before you, the days of my life all prepared before I'd even lived one day.*

Psalm 139:13-16 (MSG)

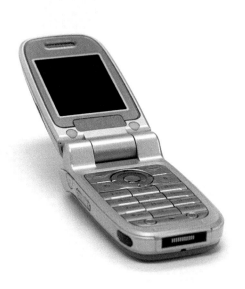

# 2

## With God All Things are Possible
### *"Even Sending a Text Message"*

*Is it possible for God to send text messages using cell phones? I guess the question sounds bizarre. If there is a God, He created everything and knows everything, so of course He could. I guess the appropriate question is whether or not God would use modern day technology to communicate with one of His children. I will reserve my opinion until the end of this chapter and let you formulate yours.*

TIME STOOD STILL as the doctor spoke to me. This would not be the last time we would get bad news. This would not be the last time that I would stand dazed and time would cease to exist.

The doctor had not seen the ultrasound results. She had merely received a report from the nurse via the phone. Nevertheless, she had to tell us what had been seen.

The doctor informed me that there were major problems with the brain, heart, and lungs. She could not tell us more than that because she had not actually seen the results. Also, the machine that they used was not top-notch. It was a little blurry. It suited their regular purposes, but was not able to see more in cases like ours.

I told my wife what the doctor said. She was holding herself together, but barely. The nurse told us that they had made another appointment for the following day in a doctor's office that had better equipment. We agreed to go, and then left.

We made two steps outside the door before my wife cracked and started to cry. I immediately hugged her and wept with her. After a few moments, we gathered ourselves and went to the car.

I decided to call back our family and relatives and ask them to pray. I also sent text messages to those two girls. I will try to explain the oddity that occurred when I sent those text messages.

My phone had a program that would attempt to complete words for you while sending text messages. For example, if I typed in the letters "th," it might type in "ough" for me in faded print and I could accept it if it was the word I desired.

When I typed the text messages, twice the program tried to complete words for me. Both times I typed "the." Both times the program attempted to complete the word with "prayer." It was odd because it would not even form a word. I thought maybe it was a glitch and even tried to get my phone to duplicate this feat, but I was unsuccessful.

I admit it could have been a glitch. Regardless of how it arrived, I now believe that God Himself sent that text message. I believe that He was telling me that I needed to talk to Him to get through what lied ahead.

My wife and I went home. We talked quite a bit. We didn't want to believe any of it. Their machine was blurry. It could have been wrong, right? We would find out tomorrow.

> *Jesus looked at them and said, "With*
> *man this is impossible, but not with*
> *God; all things are possible with God."*
> -Mark 10:27 (NIV)

✝✝✝

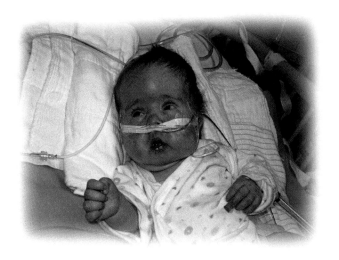

*Bella*

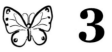

# 3

## We Wanted a Quick Fix

*Our society is one that is fast-paced. We want what we want and we want it yesterday. We have fast food and love our remote controls. So it's no wonder that when we are faced with a crisis, all we want is our comfort restored, and we want it quickly. This was definitely my state of mind at this point in the process. I wanted a one-time, super-quick miracle so I would not have to go through any hardship. I don't know what you are currently going through, but I suggest that you dig your heels in and decide that you will be patient and keep hoping at the same time. You should learn all you can about life and God through the circumstances that you are currently in.*

THE NEXT MORNING, after little sleep, we went to see our second doctor. There would be countless others, but this was the first one who would give us some specifics into our daughter's pain.

We had our second ultrasound in two days. This machine was better. We saw more. At the end of the exam, we went to meet the doctor in his office. We still hoped for the best.

When we sat down with the doctor, he told us that we had a major problem. Our daughter had spina bifida. The first thing that he mentioned was that it was not too late to legally terminate the pregnancy. The look in his eyes told me that he considered that option to be the humane one with regards to my girl.

We told the doctor that termination was not an option for us. That was the truth. No matter what the doctors told us, my wife and I never even discussed the option of abortion. It was our little girl and we did not want to hurt her.

He then gave us a different recommendation. He suggested that we go through a procedure called amniocentesis. He would stick a needle into my wife's belly and draw out some amniotic fluid so it could be tested.

I would have consented but the doctor informed me that there was a three percent chance that the baby would die. I asked him what the function of the procedure was. He said it would determine if the baby had any other complications such as Downs Syndrome. I told him that we would not undergo the procedure if the only purpose were to determine if she had something that he couldn't help anyway.

The last suggestion the doctor had was to check out a hospital in Philadelphia. This hospital was doing experimental surgery on babies with spina bifida. They actually removed the baby and repaired the spine while it was still in the womb. The mom would then carry the baby to term. We told him we would check it out.

He finished by explaining what everything meant. Our daughter's spine did not close all the way down. It kind of looked like a zipper that was open at the bottom. Due to that, the spinal cord had grown outside of the back, which hadn't closed all the way. This also caused a significant amount of water to be still present in her brain, since it had no outlet.

The doctor informed us that the extent of the damage would correlate to the spot in the spine where the spine was open from. He could not tell exactly where Bella's problem started, but it seemed pretty bad. He told us that he thought that there would be a 25 percent chance that she would never walk, a 25 percent chance that she would not be able to use the bathroom properly, and the same chance that she would be mentally retarded.

The doctor referred us to another doctor, who was a specialist with spine injuries, and who also had a better ultrasound machine. The appointment would wait a bit because that night we left to chaperone the school trip.

As we walked out of the doctor's office, we wept.

*Even when the way goes through Death*
*Valley, I'm not afraid when you walk at*
*my side.*
-Psalm 23:4 (MSG)

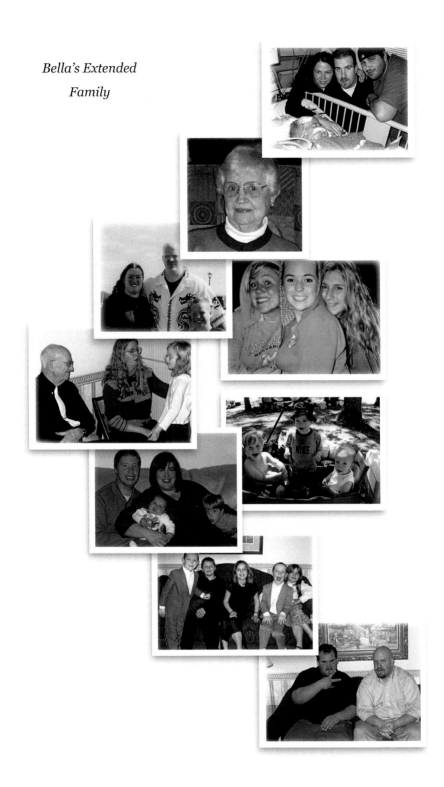

*Bella's Extended Family*

# 4

## Don't Go It Alone

*More than likely, you are not the only one who has gone, or will go, through what you are currently going through. I've found that it helps to have people involved in the situation. I'm not insinuating that you have to tell everyone, only that you should tell someone. I believe that sharing will help you. If you handle your situation well, it will also help others in the long run.*

My WIFE AND I left that night to chaperone the senior trip. We were definitely not in the mood to be around 25 overly-excited 17 year olds. We did not want to be depressed or sad and ruin their trip for them. At the same time, we thought we would inform the class of what was going on.

The reason we thought we would share our personal life with them has to do with a lesson I taught them in their eleventh grade Bible class. The class was designed to prepare them to defend their faith in Jesus.

One day the topic of discussion was to be faith. I had the class write down everything that they believed necessary in order to have a miracle happen. Some said that you just had to believe and it would occur. Others said you must believe and ask God. Others said that God must desire it to happen as well.

I informed them that they were all talk. They did not believe what they said they believed. I told them of a story that I had heard of a college professor who started off his evolution class with an egg in his hand.

This professor would tell his class that he would offend all of his Christian students that semester, but that he didn't care. He didn't care because he was right, and they were wrong. He told them he would challenge them to prove it.

He told the class that if they really believed in God and miracles then they could stand up in front of everyone and ask God for one.

The professor was going to roll an egg off his countertop and gravity would kick in and the egg would hit the tile floor and it would crack. Anyone who believed to the contrary could stand up and make their case, and then the egg would roll.

After I told them about this story, I produced an egg. I asked them if anyone had the guts, in a Christian school, to ask God for a miracle. I told them I would drop the egg, so don't fake it. A girl in the back of the class raised her hand and said maybe I shouldn't be doing this. She felt like we were tempting God.

Much to my surprise, two girls raised their hands and said they would ask God to suspend the laws of

Physics for our experiment. They stood up and prayed to God. I was inspired that they had the guts.

After they prayed, I told them that I would not drop the egg. It was only an experiment to prove that they didn't really believe. That same girl in the back of the classroom raised her hand. She informed me that I had to drop the egg. She had to know what would happen. I did, and the egg cracked.

On the trip, I recalled using this illustration with the youth. I told them that this situation was my egg. I desperately wanted to see a miracle, and not have my egg crack. I asked them to join me in praying for a miracle.

*My theme song is God's love and justice,*
*and I'm singing it right to you, God.*
*I'm finding my way down the road of*
*right living, but how long before you*
*show up? I'm doing the very best I*
*can, And I'm doing it at home, where it*
*counts.*
*Psalm 101:1 (MSG)*

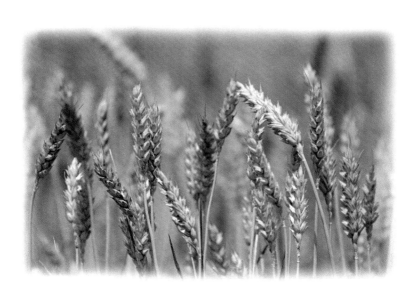

# Separating the Wheat from the Chaff

*Combining the truth about what is happening in the natural scientifically and still having faith in what God has promised you are tough lines to stay on the correct side of. Someone who had been through some tough times with his child gave me some sound advice, and I pass it on to you. Get the information. You can even have doctors tell you what the symptoms have meant in the past. Draw the line and actually ask doctors to not tell you what it means in the future for your specific instance. They do not know the future. They are wrong as often as weathermen. Certainly they will not take into account divine intervention. So ask them what is going on, what it's meant in the past, and leave it at that.*

RIGHT AFTER WE got home from the trip, we went to our third ultrasound. This would be far more thorough. This would see everything. All questions would be answered.

The ultrasound equipment they used was cutting edge. It was experimental. It was also incredible.

The equipment displayed images in 4-D. It had height, depth, width, and was displayed in time. If you don't understand what I mean, it was a computer-simulated 3-D model of our daughter. We actually watched her drink in the womb! We could see everything, including what she looked like.

The process took over seven hours that day. Over four hours of ultrasound, and three hours of waiting and moving around. At the end of the day, we were tired and still had not heard any results.

At that point, we sat with the doctor. She looked solemn. The news was worse than anything we had heard yet.

She asked if we had considered terminating the pregnancy. We told her it was not an option. She then told us that the clinic in Philadelphia was no longer an option. They only took children with spina bifida. Bella had that, but also had other issues that excluded her as a potential patient.

She had spina bifida. She had water on the brain. She had no spleen. She had only one kidney. She didn't have the vein that returned blood to the heart, although her body had compensated for that.

It was one thing to know this information. But I didn't know what it meant. I asked the doctor what it all meant; how it would play out.

The doctor told us that there was a 60 percent chance that our daughter would live to be born. If she lived, she would have brain damage of some sort and would be a paraplegic. She would not be able to control her bladder either.

We sat in shock. We did not talk. We then walked down the hall and got in the elevator. We went outside and broke down together.

> *He's God, our God, in charge of the*
> *whole earth.  And he remembers,*
> *remembers his Covenant— for a*
> *thousand generations he's been as good*
> *as his Word.*
> *-Psalm 105:7 (MSG)*

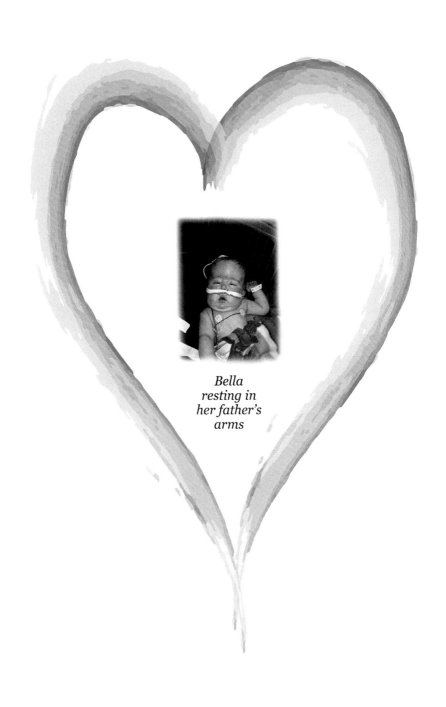

*Bella
resting in
her father's
arms*

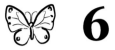

# Getting to Know God's Heart

*From the onset of our trouble, I decided my goal was to get to know God's heart on matters. A key ingredient in doing that was prayer. I held a couple of prayer meetings at my house and constantly talked to God. Prayer, when done the way God prescribes, has a profound effect on things.*

FROM THE INITIAL ultrasound with Dr. Treadwell until Bella's birthday, September 30th, there were no significant changes. On September 29th, I wrote in a journal about what I was thinking and feeling. I honestly didn't know what to expect. I wrote that I thought she would be born alive and that somehow I thought she would be able to move her feet.

We arrived to the hospital early. We got checked into a room. They prepped my wife for surgery. We made small talk with the hospital staff, but really there was an air of anticipation that was all I could hear.

They came to our room and we left to go have the C-section. We arrived at a freezing cold operating room. Many people were there, including medical students. This case was an anomaly, so many wanted to see what would happen.

It was strange to see doctors operate on my wife. She didn't feel anything and would ask me what was going on. I would tell her that they were cutting her open, and she would ask, "Really?"

The moment arrived. They pulled my daughter out. I was still seated. They wrapped her whole body in a towel and passed her in the towel to the other doctors who were baby specialists. We didn't see her very well. We did not know if she was alive. We just stared. And hoped. And waited.

Time had taken on a new dimension. It had slowed down. We were watching the scene unfold a frame at a time. Even though there was a lot of noise, we heard none of it. There was a deafening silence.

Then I heard the most wonderful noise. Isabella cried. She was alive. I immediately started crying. I fell in love with her instantaneously. In one sense, I no longer cared if she walked. I would do whatever I needed to do to help this child. If I needed to build ramps, carry her everywhere, go easy on her, or be tough on her, I could and would do it. I loved her and would give all that I had to her.

*I will give you the keys of the kingdom*
*of heaven; whatever*
*you bind on earth will be bound in*
*heaven, and whatever you loose on*
*earth will be loosed in heaven.*
*- Matthew 16:19 (NIV)*

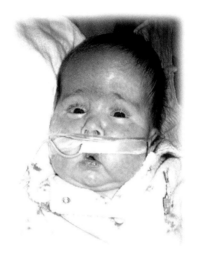

*Bella*

# 7

## God of Miracles

*God is still a God of miracles. I grant you that I don't understand all there is to know about them, but I know what I know. I can't deny what I've seen. God created the laws of the universe and from time to time likes to show us that He supercedes them. I know this not because I've studied miracles, but because I have seen something that science cannot explain.*

THE DOCTORS TOOK some measurements, cleaned her up, and then brought her to us so we could see her before they took her to get her ready for surgery. It is hard to describe what I saw because I saw her through the eyes of a father. She was the most beautiful girl I'd ever seen. Objectively speaking, her head was very large. It was probably twice the size it should have been.

They took Bella away to observe her and get her ready for surgery while I stayed with my wife. We went to a recovery room and I went to get our parents to tell them what was going on. People took turns visiting with Shelby while I found out what was going on with Bella.

Bella was in a room and no one was allowed in, including me. However, there was an observation window that people could look at her through. I went and started bringing visitors to see her through that window. Grandparents got to go first. Then I took down some other family members and friends. On a special note, three members of our youth group: Caroline Jungquist, Kayleigh Lemon, and Velita Martin got permission from their parents to skip school so they could come support us on this special day. Their love and support on this crucial day in our lives will forever be remembered and appreciated.

Eventually, they let me in. I took in a video camera and filmed her. I then talked to the doctor who had been studying her. He confirmed that she had no response from the waist down. It didn't affect me. I was okay with it. I told my mom, who was standing in the hallway, what the doctor had said. She went back to the waiting room and told the other three grandparents what had been said.

The grandparents collectively said that her not being able to move was unacceptable. They huddled together in the middle of the waiting room and asked God to do the impossible. They wanted her to be able to move.

Meanwhile, I was alone with my daughter. The team from Children's Hospital showed up to take us to surgery. The lady asked if I had seen Bella's back. I said no. She asked if I wanted to. I hesitated, and then said yes.

Her back was a large, open wound. The opening was diamond-shaped and went from her shoulder blades down to her butt. Her spinal cord was growing outside of her back. I looked, and then got out of their way.

Then, the most interesting thing happened. The lady who had come to get Bella said that she saw a great sign. I asked her what she saw. She said that Bella was moving her feet. I moved closer and watched for myself. Sure enough, her feet were moving and she was controlling them.

I must reiterate at this time that her spinal cord, which would have sent the signal from her brain to her feet, was outside of her body. I believe that I may be one of the only people ever to witness something of this magnitude. I began to sob.

I heard God whisper directly into my heart, "I will do far more than you could ever hope or dream."

*I pray that out of his glorious riches*
*he may strengthen you with power*
*through his Spirit in your inner being,*
*so that Christ may dwell in your hearts*
*through faith. And I pray that you,*
*being rooted and established in love,*
*may have power, together with all the*
*saints, to grasp how wide and long*

*and high and deep is the love of Christ,*
*and to know this love that surpasses*
*knowledge—that you may be filled*
*to the measure of all the fullness of*
*God. Now to him who is able to do*
*immeasurably more than all we ask or*
*imagine, according to his power that is*
*at work within us, to him be glory in the*
*church and in Christ Jesus throughout*
*all generations, for ever and ever!*
*Amen.*
*-Ephesians 3:16-21 (NIV)*

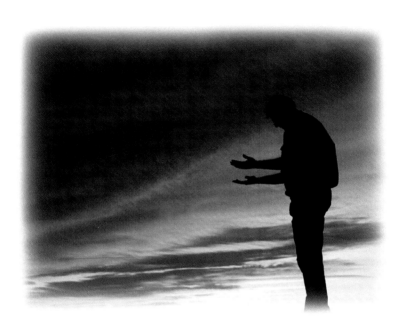

# 8

## Alone...But Not Alone

*Sometimes when you are going through something, you feel alone. Several times on Bella's birthday, I was kind of alone. During the surgery, my wife was medicated, so to some degree I was alone. When I rode with the ambulance, there were people there, but I was alone. Sitting in the NICU with my girl, I was alone. Despite these times, I knew that day that I was never totally alone. God made sure, through circumstances, and in other ways in which He was almost tangible, that He was going through this with me. His name is Emmanuel, which means "God with us." On Bella's birthday, I came to really understand that He was with me.*

BELLA AND I went with the people from Children's Hospital to ride in an ambulance to the other hospital. An underground tunnel connected the two hospitals, but the doctors said riding in an ambulance was more sterile.

I sat and stared at my daughter. I watched her feet move again and again. I couldn't stop crying. Everything was so surreal. It was as if I were still watching a movie.

After a few short minutes, we arrived at Children's.

There are a couple of things that I remember about this point in time. One memory is of a nurse. Her name was Marcie.

She saw that I was crying, and I assume that she thought it was for bad reasons. She brought me some tissue. What I found to be significant about it was the manner in which she gave it to me. She gave me the tissue discretely. She slipped it into my hand from behind so no one could see. She did not say anything to me, nor did anyone see what she had done. I had never experienced anyone who was so considerate of how someone else might be feeling. I will never forget how far a simple act of sincere kindness can go.

Bella and I did not have our own room. The room we were in could fit six babies, and I believe there were five in there on that day. The baby boy next to Bella was in the midst of a ceremony. They called it a baptism, and depending on what your religious affiliation is, you might call it a baby dedication. The boy did not appear to be doing well.

One last thing I remember about that moment in time was a teddy bear in the crib next to Bella's. I was seriously bothered by the fact that I had not been thoughtful enough to get my daughter a teddy bear. I vowed in my heart that as soon as opportunity presented itself, I would get my daughter the best teddy bear, and not one that I had conveniently bought from the hospital gift shop.

A little while later, the doctors came to get Bella for her surgery. We went to a different floor and waited in a pre-operation room. I gave the doctors the consent they needed and they told me the surgery was to close up Bella's back. While waiting, a different nurse came to speak with me. She told me that she thought that Bella needed a teddy bear and handed me one. I began to weep again. It would seem that God cared about every detail of my life.

After a couple hours, they returned to tell me the surgery went well. There was going to be another surgery on Monday (she was born on Friday) and then she could go home. That was it. End of story. She would walk, talk, and do everything normal kids did. The impossible had happened. We had won. Everything would be perfect from now on.

Or so we thought.

> *...Be content with what you have,*
> *because God has said,*
> *"Never will I leave you; never will I*
> *forsake you."*
> *So we say with confidence,*
> *"The Lord is my helper; I will not be*
> *afraid. What can man do to me?"*
> *-Hebrews 13:5, 6 (NIV)*

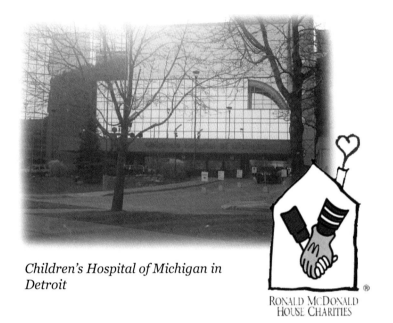

*Children's Hospital of Michigan in Detroit*

RONALD McDONALD
HOUSE CHARITIES
®

# 9

## Serving Others – the Ronald McDonald House

*I believe that to be fulfilled in life, one of the things you must do is serve other people. Selfish people never seem satisfied. They are always trying to improve their own comfort level. If you've ever met anyone who gave of themselves to help others, they always seem more fulfilled. One organization that truly serves others is the Ronald McDonald house.*

THAT NIGHT WE stayed at the hospital. My wife had a room at the hospital that she had Bella in. I was exhausted. I could not sleep. When I would doze off, I would awaken and find that I had been crying in my sleep. I found myself thanking God constantly. By five a.m., I had had enough. I needed to see my girl. My wife wanted to go with me. I wheeled her through the tunnel to see Bella.

The weekend was uneventful. My wife recovered quickly. On Monday, we both went to kiss our girl prior to her surgery and then on to the waiting room. In this surgery, the doctor would insert a tube into her head that would allow the extra spinal fluid to drain into her stomach cavity. The surgery went off without a hitch. The doctors decided to keep Bella until they were sure she could eat and breathe without difficulty. We would wait a couple more days. My wife's insurance would not pay for any more time at the hospital, so we moved into the Ronald McDonald House. I'd like to describe the ministry that goes on there and encourage you to support it whenever you can.

The Ronald McDonald House is similar to a hotel that is available to parents who have a child at the hospital. It was in the parking lot of the hospital. The rent was only $10 a night, although someone anonymously paid for our rent frequently. There is free food and drink for all who stay there, as well as free laundry. They have a play area for children and rooms to watch television or movies.

The whole operation revolves around a desperate need that people have. Recognizing that need, the operation tries hard to fill any needs that parents have: physical, spiritual, social, or emotional. Personally, I will never forget the help that was afforded me through this ministry.

*Whoever wants to be great must*
*become a servant.*
*Whoever wants to be first among you*
*must be your slave. That is what the*

*Son of Man has done: He came to serve,*
*not be served—and then to give away*
*his life in exchange for the many who*
*are held hostage.*
*-Matthew 20:28 (MSG)*

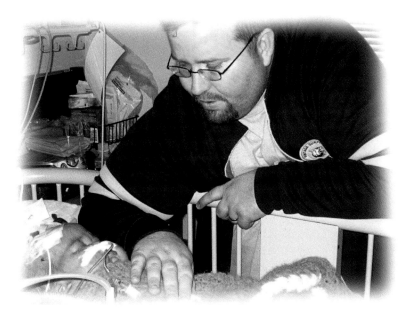

*Bella and Buddy (Allen) Shuh*

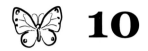

# 10

## Almost Home: *"Refusing to Give Up Hope"*

*I would like to encourage you to not lose focus. At this stage in our situation, we were told everything was miraculous and our daughter was coming home. There were only a few minor glitches. I believe it caused us to relent a little in our fervor. In our minds, the battle was over. We had won. Don't allow yourself into this place of complacency.*

WITHIN A WEEK of her birth, it seemed like Bella was coming home. But we ran into a glitch. Bella caught an infection from her neighbor. Sadly enough, it is now my experience that the hospital is the easiest place on the planet to get sick. With other sick babies in the room, it was almost inevitable. The doctors started giving her antibiotics and told us it would probably be two weeks before the infection cleared up and she could come home.

We settled into a new routine at the Ronald McDonald House. My wife stayed there while I got up early and went home to shower before work. I would drive back after work and visit with my daughter on my way back to where we were staying. My wife and I were still very excited about how well our girl was doing.

In the meantime, we began to talk with some of the other residents there. Every story seemed sadder than the previous one. There was a sorrow that dwelt there that was tangible. The only reason hope existed there was because no matter what the odds, parents refuse to give up all hope when it's their child's life that is on the line.

I actually felt guilty at times when I thought about how well Bella was doing. I remember one family telling me that they would be there for sure through Christmas. They were okay with that so long as their child survived. I couldn't imagine that. We would probably be home in a week.

Bella started to rebound from her infection about 8 days after it started. Two days later, she had a different problem. It looked like pneumonia. She probably contrived it from another infant in the nursery. This might take longer to heal up. It was pretty serious. Maybe a month and we would be home.

After about five weeks of staying at the Ronald McDonald House, my wife and I decided to move back home. Don't get me wrong; this charity was wonderful. But it was a sad place and we wanted to remain positive. In one week, three sets of parents that we knew and hung out with lost their children. It was pretty hard to bear.

At this point, one minor thing after another

seemed to happen. I recall always thinking, "she just needs to clear this thing up and she'll be home next week." Our goal now was Thanksgiving. What a perfect time to bring her home. We were having people over at my house, and we thought we'd surprise them. The call finally came. We could take her home. But it was late in the evening. We decided to bring her home when there would not be a million people there.

The next day we went to pick up our girl. We were flying high. Pure excitement. But when we got there, they told us that they had switched the oxygen she was on to vapal therm. They were waiting for approval from the insurance company because it was very expensive. They couldn't get in touch with anyone due to the holiday. Maybe we could take her home tomorrow.

The next morning Bella tested positive for an infection in her shunt (the tube in her head). They did a surgery to remove it and replaced it with a tube that would drain her spinal fluid to an external bag. They told us that they would wait until the infection cleared up and then put the shunt back in. This could be anywhere from a couple of days to a couple of weeks. Maybe she would be home for Christmas. That would be great.

On Wednesday, December 7th, my wife and I went to bed at about 10:30. A short while later, the phone rang. It was the hospital. Bella was having serious problems and they needed to operate to find out what was going on. We rushed down there.

The surgery was done at about 2:30 a.m. The doctor came and gave us the report. Her stomach had twisted itself around and actually choked off part of itself. It was dead. He had to remove that part. She had "short-gut" now. A normal baby has about 150cm of intestine. Bella now had 67 cm. The doctor told us that he believed she had enough intestines left to sustain life, but only time would tell.

We waited some more. And some more. And some more. These times were tough, physically and especially emotionally. I recall two specific instances that were tough for me. Once I was in the waiting room and I saw a large family of about 25 collectively make a decision to pull the life support plug from an infant. The grieving was intense. It was a decision that no family should ever have to make. I also remember being in Bella's room when they put up some curtains around a mother with her baby and asked us to leave the room. The mother wanted to be holding her child and looking into its eyes as it died.

At this point, I was still just waiting for the "next thing" to clear up so I could bring Bella home. I had no idea that I would personally come face to face with both situations in the previous paragraph.

*And that about wraps it up. God is*
*strong, and he wants you strong. So*
*take everything the Master has set out*

*for you, well-made weapons of the best materials. And put them to use so you will be able to stand up to everything the Devil throws your way. This is no afternoon athletic contest that we'll walk away from and forget about in a couple of hours. This is for keeps, a life-or-death fight to the finish against the Devil and all his angels.*

*-Ephesians 6:10-12 (MSG)*

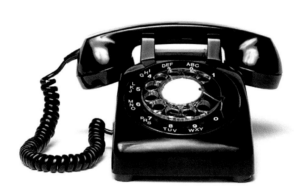

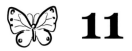

# 11

## The Phone Call

*Did you ever get a bad phone call? Did you ever freeze because the phone rang in the middle of the night and you suspected bad news? My wife and I had been called in the middle of the night before, but somehow this time seemed different.*

MARCH 5TH, 2006 was a day of great joy and laughter. It would be the last of its kind for a while. It was my son's birthday. He turned two. We joined family and close friends at a restaurant and opened his presents and had cake. It was a great day.

March 6th, 2006 ended with our regular routine. The last thing we would do before going to sleep was to call the hospital. "How's our girlie doing?" we would ask. That night she seemed to be doing a little better than she had been. She was breathing a little easier. We fell asleep about 10:30.

The phone rang at 3 a.m. It was the neuro-surgeon. She said that Bella's drain was a little clogged, and that they would do surgery to fix it at 7 in the morning. It was no big deal. Bella had already had this surgery about five times. Nevertheless, my wife and I could not fall back asleep.

We arrived at about 6 a.m. so we could spend some time with our daughter prior to her surgery. We walked with the surgery team to the elevator and kissed her goodbye. We then went to the waiting room. Maybe an hour or an hour and a half later the surgeon came out. Everything went smoothly. She'd be back in her room shortly.

My wife and I headed upstairs. We knew the drill. It would be about a half hour before we were allowed in to see her. We would wait in the waiting room on her floor.

When we went upstairs, we noticed that the waiting room was blocked off. It was being cleaned. My wife went to use the restroom. When she came out, we decided to go to the nurse's desk and see, if by some miracle, Bella was ready to have visitors yet. Amazingly enough, they let us go straight back.

When we entered the room, something was different. The surgeon was there. She was never there. She turned around and had a look of urgency in her eyes. That was something else I'd never seen. She was one of the calmest people I've ever met.

The surgeon told us that we might not want to be in there. We could stay if we wanted, but Bella was bleeding from her brain into the bag. I looked into my wife's eyes. There was no way she could stay in the room, so we went into the hallway. The hospital's chaplain came to talk with us. She opened a room for us to sit in while we waited to talk to the doctors.

A little while later, the doctors came to talk to

us. They said it was the worst-case scenario. The blood coming from her head was clotting fast. They could no longer drain it. It was just a matter of time. They said it would be anywhere between two days and two weeks. I asked them all to leave the room.

My wife and I embraced and started bawling uncontrollably.

Later, the doctors returned. We wanted to discuss what to do. They said that there nothing left for them to do. They recommended that we call family and friends to inform them and allow them to come visit one last time if they so desired.

They also said that we needed to consider pulling her off of life support. She would only live about one minute if we did, but she would not have to suffer at all. I asked if she appeared to be in pain at that time, and they said no. I decided to wait.

We called people. Many rushed to the hospital to see her and show their support of us. We cried a lot that day. We checked back into the Ronald McDonald House. We went to bed at about 10 that night. Bella actually seemed to be doing better than she had in the previous weeks.

*Jesus wept.*

-John 11:35 (NIV)

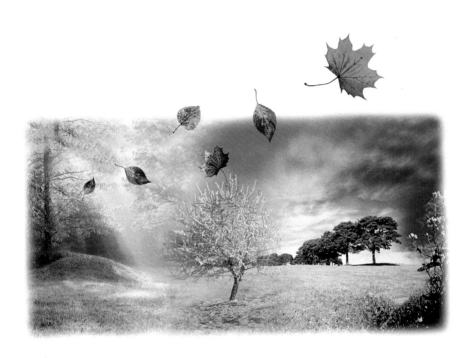

# 12

## For Everything There is a Season

*Has anyone close to you died?  It is a painful time. I think it is in that pain that you make a decision to run from God or towards Him. I do not claim to understand why my daughter died, but I decided one thing for certain: God was not at fault.  He is good and loving all the time.*

WE WERE EXHAUSTED. The emotional release from the day before was more draining than anything I'd ever gone through before.  My wife and I were still in bed when my phone went off. It was a text message.  It was a group of students from my Bible class. Their names were: Brianna Chrenko, Deborah Molnar, and Katie Folk. Ordinarily, I would have been with them at that time.  They had heard rumors and wanted to hear from me what was going on. I told them.

These three students really wanted to come see Bella. I didn't have a problem with that if the school and their parents gave them permission. Soon after, they were heading down to see us.

I got showered and got a cup of coffee while

my wife was getting ready. The three girls had texted me again, telling me that they were only a couple of miles away. They were going to meet us at the Ronald McDonald House.

My phone rang. It was Bella's nurse. She told me that I'd probably want to start heading up to her room now.

I ran to get Shelby. I sent a text message telling the girls to meet us in the waiting room on Bella's floor. We rushed over to the hospital.

The instant I stepped into Bella's room, time started doing that funny thing again. It was moving in slow motion, and I was trapped in a movie.

The very first thing I noticed was that the curtain was up all around Bella's bed. I refused to think about it, but in the back of my mind I fully understood the implication.

I came around the curtain and saw my little girl. For the first time in forever, she was not hooked up to anything electronic. I instinctively looked at the machine to see her heart rate and oxygen levels, but they were turned off. I saw her tiny chest breathe in and out.

The nurse was a bit frantic. She told my wife to hurry up and sit down if she wanted to be holding her when she passed. My wife did as she was told. The nurse was trying to unhook some tubes so she could hand Bella to my wife.

Another nurse was around the other side of

Bella's bed. She took her stethoscope and put it to Bella's chest. She looked at the other nurse and shook her head from side to side. I couldn't swallow. I found it hard to breathe.

I looked at my wife and knew that she hadn't seen the nurse's reaction. She was still waiting to hold Bella. My wife looked at me and knew something was wrong. She asked me if Bella was still alive. I told her no. She was gone.

We both started sobbing. The nurse continued what she was doing and then handed my wife our daughter's body. She cradled it and started rocking while bawling out of control. I was kneeling on the floor next to the rocking chair. I had my arms around both of them. We sat like this for a few minutes, just crying out of control.

*When the perishable has been clothed*
*with the imperishable, and the mortal*
*with immortality, then the saying*
*that is written will come true: "Death*
*has been swallowed up in victory."*
*"Where, O death is your victory?*
*Where, O death is your sting?" The*
*sting of death is sin, and the power of*
*sin is the law. But thanks be to God!*
*He gives us the victory through our*
*Lord Jesus Christ. Therefore, my dear*

*brothers, stand firm. Let nothing move you. Always give yourselves fully to the work of the Lord, because you know that your labor in the Lord is not in vain.*

-I Corinthians 15:54-58 (NIV)

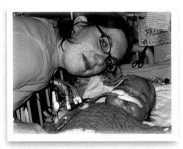

*Mommy (Shelby Shuh) and Bella*

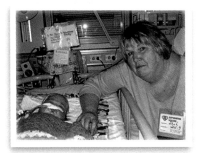

*Grandma Martin and Bella*

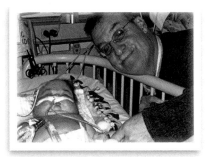

*Papa Martin*

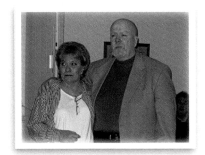

*Grandma and Papa Shuh*

# 13

## Aftermath

*In the midst of your pain, don't neglect to see the positive. With Bella's death came some of the sweetest times of my life. Although it was the most painful thing I've ever experienced, I've never experienced more real love from friends and family.*

THE PAIN WAS immense. My brain started to go into overdrive. In retrospect, I think my brain started to go through the mechanics of what needed to happen now because I couldn't take was happening. I needed something to do. I asked the nurse what was going to happen now.

She told me that a lot of parents like to bathe the child and then dress it. That was about the last thing that I wanted to do. I didn't understand. The nurse said that it sometimes helped the parents. I declined, but my wife wanted to do that. We decided that while she was doing that, I would call people and inform them of what had happened.

The hospital opened up a medium sized conference room for us. They said that some family would probably like to come down and see Bella one last time. I went to the conference room and turned my cell phone back on. I had several text messages and voicemails waiting for me.

I read the text messages. One was from Brianna, who was now in the waiting room. I decided to text the news to her so they would have a moment to ingest the news before seeing me. I then listened to my voicemails.

The first person I called was my father-in-law. I was not hysterical when I dialed the number. But as I tried to speak, I found that I could not. Words were replaced with sobs. He asked if everything was okay. He was already crying. I told him no. Finally, I told him she was gone. He was crying as I heard him tell his wife. She erupted in a painful, screaming type of cry. He said they would leave right then.

I then called my parents and had about the same reaction. I figured that the two sets of grandparents would tell the rest of the family. I also called the associate pastor of my church. He said he'd come down as well.

I went out to see the three girls in the waiting room. When I came around the corner, they stood up. They were a wreck. They gave me a hug and we sat down. A hospital worker offered to go get the chaplain. I told him that I had already talked to her. We sat for a moment and then another family friend, Sheri Bucher, showed up. I told her what happened. We cried some more. We then all went back to the conference room.

I went back to see my wife. The bath was done and I helped her get Bella dressed. The nurse said that most parents would take her into the conference room so the family could see her. I wasn't sure I wanted to do that. But I realized that I knew little about grieving and these types of situations, so I decided to take the nurse's advice.

We sat in the conference room. When a family member or friend showed up, my wife and I would go to them and hug. Inevitably, there was a lot of crying. Then things would cool down and people would talk. The cycle would repeat every time someone new showed up. I have never experienced something so emotional. It was the saddest moments of my life, and yet in the thick of it, I saw something that was equally beautiful. It was love. The love expressed in that room that day was authentic and tangible. When people would say that they loved me, it was so powerful that it actually hurt.

One last thing I remember about that day was a visitor that I did not expect. His name was Keith Valentine. We were all sitting in the conference room when a man that I had never seen asked my wife and I to step into the hallway. He told us his name and that he attended my sister-in-law's church. We had heard his story but had never met him.

Keith and his wife had been in a similar situation as ours. Their baby's brain had grown outside of the skull while in the womb. They had been told to abort, but they chose not to. Their child's surgery had gone well, and he was now a year old. They were not out of the clear yet, and had undergone a lot. Their son had had many surgeries.

Keith did not know that Bella had died. He informed us that my wife's sister had called them the previous night to update them on our situation so they could pray. They knew that the doctors had told us to think about pulling life support, and how hard of a decision that would be.

Keith told me that he had been sitting at work when he felt strongly like God wanted him to leave and come talk to us at the hospital. So he did. The doctors had told him to consider pulling life support on his child a couple of times. He cried as he told us these things.

He then told us why he had come. He wanted to share what God had told him. The decision to pull life support or not was not an indicator of your love for your child. In other words, if we decided to do it, it did not mean that we didn't love her. It would only mean that we were leaving it in God's hands.

Then Keith said what he had been sent to say. He said that Bella was God's girl. We only had her temporarily, and that we should just do what we thought best for her. Ultimately, she would go be with God anyway, so we could release her if we wanted to.

We told Keith that Bella had passed on. We also

thanked him from the bottom of our hearts. We needed to hear that she was in God's hands and in a better place. And even though he did not know why he was sent, he was obedient to God and it was very comforting to us.

> *A new command I give you: Love one another. As I have loved you, so you must love one another. By this all men will know that you are my disciples, if you love one another.*
> *-John 13:34, 35 (NIV)*

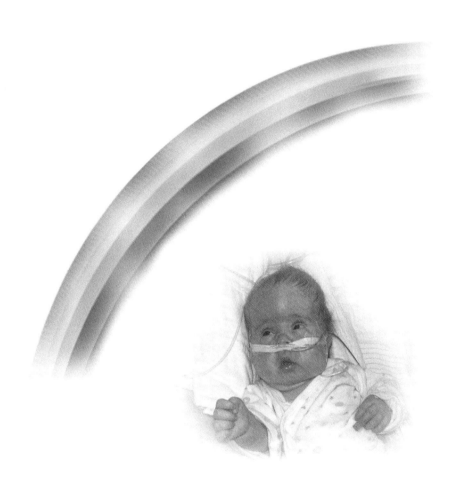

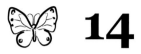

# 14

## The Home Going

*Funerals can be tremendously sad. I always use them as a time to reflect. Although we'd prefer to live a carefree life, the truth is that we will all face death someday. So I use funerals as a time of self-evaluation. Am I doing what I should? Am I doing something productive with my life? I will say one thing here: if there were no after-life, life would not have a meaning. I find hope in the fact that one day I will see Bella again. If that weren't true, I would find life meaningless.*

WE LEFT THE hospital and all went out to eat. We started discussing funeral arrangements. We decided on having a viewing on Friday night at the funeral home, and having the funeral Saturday at our church. Everyone seemed to agree that this was the best plan.

One of the sadder things that I remember was dealing with logistics in this type of circumstance. For example, my wife and I did not even have money to pay for the funeral. Thank God for my incredible family. Everyone decided to pitch in and the funeral was paid for in about a day.

There were two things that stand out to me about the viewing. The first is how many people came to support us. There were probably hundreds. Most had never met Bella, though they had prayed for her. The support was greatly appreciated. The funeral director said that he had never seen so many people show up for an infant. My family stayed all day and made sure that my wife and I didn't need anything. Also, the three girls who had been there when Bella was born (Caroline, Velita, and Kayleigh) came when the doors opened and refused to leave for the duration. I haven't seen such support and loyalty. In particular, I would like to thank a few of "my boys." A lot of people were there for us, but the next three guys were special at this time.

The first of "my boys" was Bobby Stockman. He is my armor-bearer, meaning, if I were to go to war, he'd be by my side, doing whatever I needed. At the time of the funeral, Bobby really stepped it up. He immediately volunteered to sing. He is a very talented singer, and I knew it was a sacrifice because he was hurting emotionally and would try to sing anyway. He also decided to open up his home during the viewing for all my family so we could get out for a while and eat. He provided all the food for like 30 people.

The second "boy" I'd like to recognize is my brother, Will. He is my watchman. By that, I mean he's always looking out for me. He would die for me. He always supports everything I've done, and has always been one of my best friends. During the funeral and viewing he drove us around and made sure we had everything we needed.

My third "boy" is Joel Hays. Even though we are not blood-related, he is my little brother. I asked him to be central in the speaking parts of the funeral. Not only did he do a phenomenal job at it, he also drummed for the band during songs.

The funeral was sad and poignant. Bobby sang a couple of songs. I asked another close friend, Paul Anleitner, to sing another song. Our pastors gave a eulogy. Some people also wrote things that we read at the funeral.

Kelley Hays, who is so close to our family that we consider her family, wrote a poem that her brother, Joel, read. It was written after having a dream in which she believes she saw Bella, our unborn daughter at the time...

## *Bella*

I dreamed one night
and you were there
You had bright blue eyes
With your long brown hair
And I saw that you were laughing

Baby buggy
And you jumped out

Your mom stood crying
As you walked about
And you looked at her and smiled
Your dad sat close
And watched you run
Over to him
With your shoes undone
And you climbed up and you hugged him
Then you told him that you loved him

I see you now
Tubes in your head
With drowsy blue eyes
In a hospital bed
And I wish that you were laughing

You fight so hard
To stay alive
And we watch you grow
As we pray and cry
And imagine that you smiled

I think of you
Walking with me
As I tell you the things
That I saw in my dream
And I hold you and I hug you
And I tell you that I love you

My mother-in-law was saddened by the fact that my son Isaac never met his sister, so she wrote a letter from him to Bella. My brother-in-law Adam read that one...

Hi Bella:

I'm your big brother, Isaac. I'm 2. I can put on my own socks and I'm learning to say new words every day, although Mom and Dad and others don't always know what I'm saying.

I learned to say "baby" long before you were born, when Mommy's belly got really BIG. I was at the hospital when you were born. There were lots of tears and lots of rejoicing and I knew I had a beautiful baby sister ... some thought you looked like me!

During the past 5 months, I've learned to say BELLA really good. I've had a great time being cared for by loving friends and family. I got to play at the Ronald McDonald House and learned to run up and down the ramp at Children's Hospital. I got rides in wagons and on elevators and loved being loved by so many.

Hugs and kisses are great, aren't they?

I'm sorry the hospital's and doctors' silly rules kept me from seeing you, but you will always be my beloved baby sister. One day soon we'll have our time to play and we won't ever have to stop to take a nap or clean up the mess.

Make sure you ask God about Elmo. He's pretty cool and I'm sure He's got a few up there to play with.

I love you,
*Isaac*

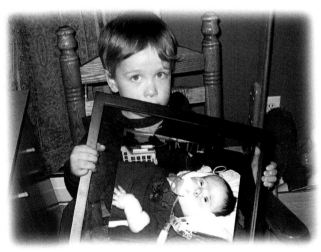

*Isaac holding a picture of Bella*

My mother wrote a story about the fact that babies are giants in heaven and she read it herself...

## *Giants of Paradise*

*It came to pass that after 92 years on earth a man died and went to heaven. He was greeted by the Master at the beginning of his new journey with a long awaited embrace.*

*The Lord took his hand and proceeded to show him the heavenly city. They walked on streets of the purest gold. The buildings were adorned with flawless diamonds and rubies. The saints wore garments made of the finest threads. The man saw some people preparing for the banquet, some creating beautiful sculptures and works of art, and some playing instruments and singing glorious songs – the sound of which his ear had never before heard. But above all, he saw some saints that appeared to be very large in stature and noticed they were the leaders of many souls. Looking closely, he saw that they had very young faces, some as young as newborn babies. They were children!*

*Curious, he asked Jesus, "Why are these children so big?"*

*He smiled and replied, "All the children are."*

*"But why?" the man asked.*

*"All children have spirits that dwarf an adult's," He answered.*

*The man was puzzled. "I don't understand."*

The Master replied, "The enemy destroyed their young bodies on earth, but he could not destroy their spirits. Satan had very little time to influence them. Therefore, their minds and hearts never shrank from doubt and unbelief."

"Do they have special titles?" the man asked.

"No," the Lord replied. "That's what makes them so special. They never placed themselves above anybody else."

"What should I call them?" the man asked.

"Call them by their names," He said, pointing at a couple of little boys. "Over there is Willie and Charlie." They started jumping up and down when they saw Him and blew him kisses. He jumped up and caught them and gave them right back.

A chubby cheeked little girl came up to Him and held out her arms. He picked her up and twirled her around while she laughed and giggled. She settled down into his arms and He held her tight as she planted little kisses on His face while she hugged His neck. "This extraordinary little girl is Isabella," He said.

The man saw the enjoyment his Master was having with these children. He said, "They're very special to you, aren't they?"

A smile spread across His face and delight danced in His eyes. "Yes, they are," He replied. "They're the giants of paradise for as such is the kingdom of heaven."

My sister read a cute poem that used the alphabet to give adjectives. I also wrote a letter of thanks that I had Joel read.

After the funeral, we drove to the cemetery. We had a short service there where Bobby sang another song. We said goodbye to Bella one last time. We then went back to the church where lunch was waiting.

One other thing that was discussed at the funeral was the "park bench." The story behind it is a little bit intricate, so I thought I would devote the next chapter to that story.

*Brothers, we do not want you to be*
*ignorant about those who fall asleep, or*
*to grieve like the rest of men, who have*
*no hope. We believe that Jesus died and*
*rose again and so we believe that God*
*will bring with Jesus those who have*
*fallen asleep in him.*
*-I Thessalonians 4:13, 14 (NIV)*

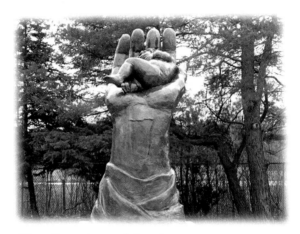

*View from the park bench*

# 15

## God knows us Better Than We Know Ourselves: *"The Park Bench"*

*I believe God knows us better than we know ourselves, and when He talks to us, He does it in a way that we will best hear Him. I love puzzles and riddles, so I believe that sometimes God leaves me signs that, in due time, become poignant messages.*

MY FAMILY HAS a close bond with the Hays' family. It was not uncommon for us to share what was going on in our lives. So it happened that about 7 years after my wife and I got married, she still was not pregnant. We had been trying for 5 of those years. So we shared with them what was going on.

One night, Kelley had a dream. It was about our child. It was a boy. He had blond hair and blue eyes. She told us about it. She said it seemed more like reality than a dream. A short while later, we were pregnant. We had a boy. A blonde, blue-eyed boy.

When we first heard the bad news from the ultrasound, the Hays were among the first to find out. Kelley was devastated. She had another dream.

In the dream, she was pushing Bella in a stroller through the park. She stopped by a park bench. Bella leapt out and ran to the bench where was presumably me.

Around Christmas time, our school does a special Christmas chapel. The idea is that it's Jesus' birthday and you bring a gift. Kayleigh decided to give a painting. It was a park bench with a girl and a man on it. At this time, she did not know about Kelley's dream. Honestly, I didn't even remember it at that time. I thought the picture was Kayleigh on the bench with Jesus.

The day before the funeral, I put the two together. They had seen the same park bench. But I didn't get it fully. Until later that day. I went to see the plot of land where Bella would be buried. Right in front of the grave sight was a monument. It was a giant hand coming out of the ground holding a small infant.

And there was a park bench.

I saw the bench and it started to come together. I went to the bench and sat down. From that viewpoint, I could no longer see Bella's grave. All I could see was that God had taken her up to be with Him.

It was on that park bench that I started to receive some healing and comfort.

*For instance, we know that when these*
*bodies of ours are taken down like tents*
*and folded away, they will be*
*replaced by resurrection bodies in*

*heaven—God-made, not handmade—*
*and we'll never have to relocate our*
*"tents" again.*
*-II Corinthians 5:1, 2 (MSG)*

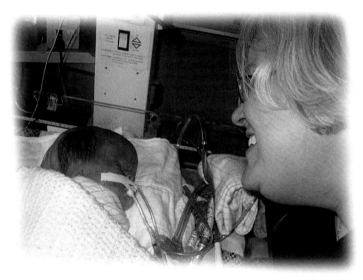

*Aunt Bonnie and three-day-old Bella*

# 16

## Miracles are Miracles
### *"Not Just Extreme Coincidences"*

*I heard it once described that sometimes a miracle could be explained away by strange circumstances, but sometimes you know, if only by the timing that the circumstance happened, that it was a miracle and that it was just for you. This chapter describes some of those things that have happened in my life.*

After the funeral, there were many strange coincidences. Jennifer Thomas is a member of our church. She and her family are some of the most wonderful people my wife and I have ever met. Shortly after the funeral, they were in a mall and saw something at Mrs. Field's that caught their attention. In the display case was a huge cookie with a cross in the middle and it said, "God bless Isabella." There were other coincidences, but none stranger than the show "Extreme Home Makeover."

I teach Bible at a Christian school. So I was excited when I saw that "The Gospel of Judas" was going to be on TV. I wanted to see if it had any merit. It

began at 8 pm. At the first commercial break, I flipped
channels. I went to "Extreme Home Makeover." It was
still the beginning of the show where the family is telling
their story.

The family had lost their son at an early age. This
immediately caught my wife's attention. I did not know
if we should watch the rest, but my wife was adamant
that we would watch it. I said okay.

Not only did this family lose a small boy, but their
next pregnancy had problems as well. They discovered
during the pregnancy that their daughter's ventricle
had not developed properly. They then showed their
daughter on her actual birthday. My wife and I froze in
our seats. It could have been our daughter's identical
twin. It appeared as if they had taken our photo from
home and put it on TV. My wife turned and looked at
me. She had a look of disbelief on her face.

As the family continued with their story,
the father became a bit emotional. He said that he
remembered the day that he brought Bella home. They
had named her Isabella, but called her by her nickname
Bella. My wife and I sat hypnotized by the show. We
were both crying uncontrollably.

The story continued. The wife was not able to
work because she was taking care of Bella. They had large
medical expenses. They were falling behind because the
father did not earn a ton of money. He was a teacher
and a coach who was heavily involved with youth. FYI:

I am a teacher and a coach and the youth leader at my church.

My wife went online to read more about this family. We also learned that they found out that they were getting their home makeover at the same time that we lost our Bella. Now I must tell you that I'm not a big believer in coincidences. The quantity and oddity of these happenings made me believe they were not random at all. I started trying to figure out what this all could mean. I think I get it.

It's another park bench. It's a confirmation of the same story. I believe that God was telling me that Bella was still alive. I am not in denial that my girl passed away, but God was telling me that only her body died. The real Bella, the one that I had fallen in love with, was alive and well and with God.

*For my thoughts are not your thoughts,*
*neither are your ways My ways," saith*
*the Lord.*
*-Isaiah 55:8 (NKJV)*

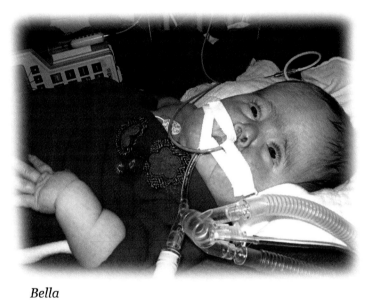

*Bella*

# 17

## Bella's Chapel

*One thing I decided to do was to talk about what had happened. I did this for several reasons. First, I did not want to pretend that Bella did not exist. I also wanted her life to be able to positively impact other people even though she had passed away. I found that in talking, I also found some healing for myself.*

AT THE SCHOOL that I teach at, I am also in charge of the chapel services. The students at the school had been very supportive of me throughout my ordeal. But I knew they had questions. If Mr. Shuh lives for God, and this happens to him, how could there really be a God? Questions like that. I knew that before the end of the year I needed to talk in chapel and explain things.

It was extremely difficult. I sat on a stool in front of 100 youth and shared pretty much everything I've written about in this book. I wept pretty much through the whole thing. It took me about an hour to get through it.

At the end of the chapel, we offered prayer. The response was big. Six youth asked Jesus to be their

Lord and Savior. Many more recommitted their lives to Christ.

Even though none of the youth had ever experienced what I had, they still connected with the "I've been hurt" aspect of the message. And they wanted to pray to get through their hurts. Probably 75 youth came forward for prayer in this area.

We had something special set up for this prayer time. Samantha Bucher, one of our other outstanding youth, had come up with this idea. We had a helium tank and balloons. The youth wrote their pain on a piece of paper and put it in the balloon. We blew up the balloon. They then went outside, asked God to help them release their hurts, and when they were ready, released the balloon.

One young girl named Katelin Wallace had lost her father that same year to a heart attack. It had been really hard on her, as you could imagine. I saw her praying and then her eyes started frantically looking around. I knew she was looking for me. She asked me to pray with her. We prayed, and held hands as she released her balloon. She then told me that she knew how busy I was, but would really like it if I could spend an hour with her on father's day. My heart melted.

A lot of positive things happened that day. You may wonder why I write about this experience when it is obviously painful. I think it would be what Bella would have wanted. Her life is helping others even after she is gone.

*Nevertheless I tell you the truth: It is
expedient for you that I go away: for
if I go not away, the Comforter will not
come unto you: but if I depart, I will
send him unto you.*
*-John 16:7 (NKJV)*

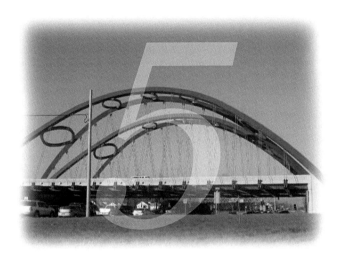

*The "large, blue bridge" in Taylor, Michigan*

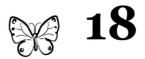

# 18

## Five Blue

*I will conclude this book with a solved riddle, one that I believe God drew my attention to, and had to explain. You may be wondering what my thoughts toward God are now. You may be wondering how you could know God in a personal way. I intend to share my answer to both those questions in this chapter.*

T HE FIRST TIME we traveled to Detroit to get what was our third ultrasound, the city of Taylor was putting in a large, blue bridge. We were actually diverted off the highway while they were doing construction. My wife and I both noticed it and she asked me what it was. I told her it was a bridge. She asked me if that meant we would ride up the big arches to get over. I cracked up. I told her it wasn't a roller coaster. We would drive through flat and the arches were either decorative or supportive of the weight.

By the next time we traveled downtown, the bridge was in and functional. I kidded my wife as I drove over it. It became a standing joke. Every time we went over it (we would travel over it many times), we would yell like we were on a roller coaster. We were always curious about the design and the strange blue color.

The day Bella was born, we had packed our bags. We knew that the best-case scenario was that we would be in the hospital for the weekend. We had all our toiletries, clothes, etc. We parked in the structure and when we got out, I paid particular attention to where we were parked. We were in section five-blue. I said it to myself several times silently in the hopes that when I eventually arrived, I would recall this section.

While we were in our room awaiting the C-section, the television was on. They had it turned to the news. Oddly enough, they were doing a segment on the blue bridge in Taylor. It had been put in for the Super bowl. Detroit officials knew most visitors would use that highway, and this bridge was the first sighting of the Super bowl festivities. It had five ovals that were supposed to represent five footballs, because it was '05. It was blue because of the Detroit Lions. Five blue footballs. Again with the five blue? It seemed so odd that it lingered in my mind for months.

One day I was reading the Bible, in the book of Titus. I read something that I had read before but had always glossed over. Paul, who wrote Titus, starts by wishing him grace and peace to him in the name of Jesus. After further review, it seemed that Paul almost always started his letters off with this phrase. In my mind, something clicked. I had heard that in the Bible, when you see the number five, it is representative of God's grace. When I think of the color blue, I think of the sky, the ocean, of peace. Grace and peace. Five blue.

I now believe that God started off this situation with me by giving me the same assurances that Paul gave Titus. Grace and peace.

First, I'll talk about God's grace. God's grace is the reason that any of us can have eternal life. I think we all are aware of our shortcomings and the fact that we have messed up in life. God is aware of these things too. Rather than punish us, though, He provided a way for us to go to heaven anyway. He allowed His Son, Jesus, to come to Earth and die as punishment for the things we have done wrong. If we believe this in our heart, and confess it with our mouth, the Bible says we will be "saved." What an awesome proposition we are presented with! All we have to do to have an eternity in heaven is admit we don't deserve it on our own merit and accept Jesus' sacrifice as atonement for our wrongs. This is God's grace, and in the eternal scheme of things, it is the most important thing that exists.

But He didn't just grant me eternal life. He also tells me that I can have peace while here on Earth. This is not a guarantee that we won't have tough times. As a matter of fact, in the book of John, Jesus tells us that we will have trials while we are here. What God tells us is that it is possible, with His help, to have peace while in those storms of life. This is God's peace. So, putting it together:  grace and peace, or five blue. I believe that on the very first day of Bella's life, God was giving me two awesome promises. The first, and most important, was that regardless of the outcome, He has provided a way for Bella and me to go to Heaven for all eternity.

Secondly, He would provide what I needed throughout this trial, which was peace.  He was telling me that He loved me and would be with me now and forever.

I conclude by telling you that the same offer is available to you.  Grace and peace.  Five blue. In order for you to receive eternal life, you must only believe in your heart and confess that you receive Jesus' sacrifice for your wrong.  He desires to be in a relationship with you, so the deciding factor will be you. I hope that this book has encouraged you during your tough time and has helped you to get to know God a little better.

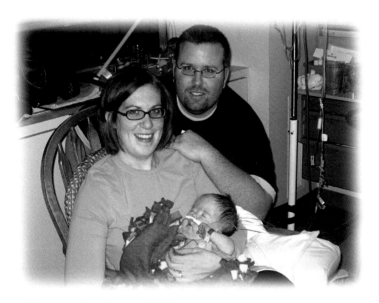

*Mommy, Daddy, and Bella*

# 19

## Thanksgiving

*This has been a rough time for us. Yet we have much to be thankful for and we wanted to acknowledge some of our thanks publicly.*

FIRST OF ALL, we give thanks to God. Father, You have been with us throughout this mess. We have felt your presence and heard your words of love. Even now, as we are walking through the valley of the shadow of death, we feel You there, loving us, guiding us, protecting us. You have been faithful even when we have not been. And of course, we are the most grateful because we know that when Bella died, You scooped her up in your loving hand and took her to heaven.

We would also like to thank our family, church, and friends. We could not have made it through this without you. We have been so distracted that at times we have neglected to even say thank you. We have the most incredible people around us and are so appreciative. I think of my grandfather, who at 84, would still literally get down on his knees to pray for Bella even though he could barely get back up. He represents how all of you have given all that you have to help us. Some of the practical ways that you have loved us are:

You gave us money. We absolutely could not have weathered this storm without your money. Shelby had to work less, and things were tight, but just when it seemed our electricity would be cut off, you would give again. The amazing thing is that we never had to ask: you just gave.

You gave gifts. For Bella, we were given a crib, dresser, rocking chair, bassinet, about 30 outfits, a handmade afghan, a handmade sterling silver bracelet with Isaac and Isabella's name on it, and bedding. The amazing thing is that we never even had a shower.

You have shown us your love in many other forms. You babysat for hundreds of hours for free. You cleaned our house and cooked for us probably 50 times. The amount of cards, hugs, and prayers that you have given us are literally uncountable.

Next, we would like to thank our youth group. You were there when she was born and you were there when she died. You were there everyday in-between. You prayed with us, and you cried with us. Bar none, we have the best youth group on the planet.

Lastly, we would like to say thanks to our beautiful daughter, Isabella Harmony Shuh. Because of you, little girl, our family is closer. Because of you, our church is a little closer. Because of you, we know God a little better. Probably the lesson that will stay with us from you is to never quit. We don't recall you ever having what we would call a "good day." Not even one day that you did not feel pain or sickness. Yet you always fought, with everything you had, to have another day. You taught us to fight for life. There is something worth living for. Never quit. Bella, we will miss you dearly but we will see you soon enough. Meet us at the park bench when we get there.

To order additional copies of *The Story of Bella*, or to find out about other books by Allen Shuh or Zoë Life Publishing, please visit our website www.zoelifepub.com.

Zoë Life Publishing
P.O. Box 871066
Canton, MI 48187
(877) 841-3400
outreach@zoelifepub.com

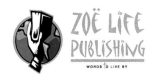